Infertility in Nigeria
Strategies for Prevention

Dr Jude Adeghe
MBBS, PhD, FRCOG.
Consultant in Gynaecology & Fertility

TABLE OF CONTENTS

About the Author

Dr Jude Adeghe is a Consultant Gynaecologist and Fertility Specialist and a successful healthcare entrepreneur.

Dr Adeghe graduated from the University of Nigeria Medical School, Enugu, Nigeria. He is a Fellow of the Royal College of Obstetricians and Gynaecologists UK (FRCOG) and also holds a PhD from the University of Birmingham, UK.

He had a distinguished career as an NHS (National Health Service) consultant in Obstetrics, Gynaecology and Assisted Reproduction for ten years before leaving the NHS to kickstart his entrepreneurial ambition. He set up his own hospital, St Jude's Women's Hospital in England, which has gone from strength to strength.

Dr Adeghe celebrated the birth of the 1000th baby from IVF service in his hospital in 2013. He is a passionate fertility clinician. Having established his practice in the United Kingdom, he is now on a mission to impact and improve fertility services in Nigeria.

DEDICATION

Dedicated to my parents who have departed
to be with the Lord, Our God:

Edward Onasere Adeghe ----- Baba
Highly intelligent and gifted MAN, the ultimate family man, Pioneer student of Edo College, Benin-City, Agriculturist & Entrepreneur.

Helen Abiona Adeghe (Nee Jegede) ---- Mama
Versatile Woman of God, multilingual, & talented Nurse & Midwife.

I am grateful for the genetic material I inherited and the immense influence on my life.

ACKNOWLEDGEMENTS

Some of the text in this book have been published previously in my women's health column in *the Authority Newspaper* in Nigeria. There are also extracts from St Jude Hospital blog, written by yours sincerely.

This year 2018 marks 40 years of successful IVF practice. The revolutionary scientific and clinical work done by Bob Edwards, Patrick Steptoe and Jean Purdy, led to the birth of the first IVF baby, Louise Brown (now Louise Mullinder) on 25th July 1978. It marked a unique milestone in fertility treatment. Since then, about 8 million babies have been born through IVF treatment. It is appropriate that I should acknowledge the efforts and brilliance of the founding fathers of IVF, something that totally captured my interest form my days in medical school. It continues to give me so much professional joy and satisfaction.

INTRODUCTION

The ability to have children represents more than a quality-of-life issue (Centers for Disease Control and Prevention. National Public Health Action Plan for the Detection, Prevention, and Management of Infertility, Atlanta, Georgia; 2014). The World Health Organisation (WHO) as well as the American Society for Reproductive Medicine, have defined infertility as a disease. It carries a huge emotional, social and financial burden and weighs heavily on both male and female partners. Further, there are credible world reports on disability indicating that Infertility in women is ranked the fifth highest serious global disability. Given that the goal of public health is to reduce disease, preventing infertility and the adverse consequences associated with its treatment are important concerns.

The prevalence of infertility in Nigeria is high and probably rising. There is significant social, emotional and financial burden inherent in infertility. The high cost of assisted conception treatments and the fact that they are not always successful are good reasons to pay attention to strategies for prevention. Many cases of infertility are preventable therefore the best way to protect one's fertility is to be educated about the risks.

This book is directed at all stakeholders in healthcare, more so at governmental policy makers and young women and men in high schools and universities, so they may become aware of the impact of some actions and lifestyles on their future fertility. Ideally this book ought to be essential reading for a short *health awareness course* in high schools.

Chapter 1
Infertility: Definition and Rationale for Prevention

The general definition of infertility is inability to conceive after 12months or more of regular unprotected sexual intercourse. Many clinicians now extend the definition to include women aged 35 years or older after 6 months of trying to conceive. Infertility is sometimes referred to as *barreness,* a severe and unfortunate term that belongs to medieval times and should have no place in modern day fertility terminology. The term "barreness" is gender-biased being almost always directed at the woman. Barreness implies a permanent state of infertility, which is often not the case. Based on better understanding of human reproductive process it is now known that many causes of infertility are relative rather than absolute. Even the absolute causes of infertility may be treatable by modern assisted conception technology. Most practitioners of fertility care would attest to the many cases of natural pregnancies that occur independent of treatment. I know many colleagues who argue that subfertility (rather than infertility) is a better descriptive term, because it reflects the "relative" nature of many causes of inability to conceive. However, the remit of this column is to inform and educate for practical benefits to the reader, so I will dwell no further on semantics.

Treatments for infertility is highly sought after by desperate couples who are often exploited by a wide range of practitioners, some of questionable calibre. The therapeutic arena is populated by witch-doctors, traditional doctors, herbalists, alternative health practitioners and medical doctors. Each group of practitioners will have a series of cases of success to justify their practice. In a country like Nigeria where there is no effective regulation of health service providers and practitioners, infertile couples are often exploited by quacks whose main motivation is the "quick naira".

The advent of reproductive technology marked by the birth of Louise Brown through In-vitro fertilisation (IVF) in 1978 offered new and genuine hope for infertile couples. By the way, Louise Brown is now herself, a mum. Since that early beginning significant progress have been made in refining the IVF process and expanding the range of assisted reproductive technology treatment options. It is now possible for couples to have babies through egg donation, through the use of surrogates, and for men with low sperm count to have treatment using a technique known as *Intracytoplasmic Sperm Injection* (ICSI) whereby a sperm either from semen or extracted surgically from the testes is injected into an egg to achieve fertilisation.

No doubt, medical science has made significant progress in alleviating the burden of infertility. However, the different treatment options offered by assisted reproductive technology are stressful, expensive and not without side effects and complications. In Nigeria where there is widespread poverty and poor healthcare facilities, IVF and other forms of fertility treatments are inaccessible and not affordable. Moreover, there is no guaranty of success with IVF, in fact the average success rate in the best clinics is at best 50% which means that around half of treatment cycles are unsuccessful.

Infertility is a good illustration of the saying that *Prevention is better and cheaper than cure*. It has to be said that some causes of infertility are self-inflicted e.g. men who are heavy smokers or drugs abusers, habits that are well known to cause sperm damage. There is a lot that individuals can do to prevent or reduce the risk of infertility. Before going on to outline preventive measures it is important to highlight common causes of infertility. Awareness of the causes of infertility will help individuals to adopt the necessary preventive measures. In fact, as one throws light upon the causes of infertility, the preventive measures become self-evident.

Chapter 2
Understanding the Causes of Infertility

In Nigeria and many other African countries, infertility affects 1 in 5 couples while in the UK it affects around in 1 in 6 couples. There are strong indications that the incidence of infertility may be rising in many parts of the world. In a recent Nigerian newspaper article, a reputable Consultant Gynaecologist in an Abuja hospital said that 60% of gynaecology clinic consultations were infertility-related. This is alarming.

Infertility is commonly blamed on the woman and it is not uncommon for the man to take on a new wife (often a younger woman) in an effort to have children. However, the fact is that the causes of infertility is equally split between male and female. 30% of cases are due to a female factor, 30% to a male factor, 30% to a combination of male and female factors, and in the remaining 10% the cause is unexplained.

Causes of Infertility

1) **Blockage of Fallopian tubes** – This is the commonest cause of infertility in Nigeria. In the UK the commonest cause of infertility is Ovulatory problems. Tubal blockage is often the consequence of Pelvic Inflammatory Disease (PID). PID may be sexually contracted or may be a complication of termination of pregnancy often carried out by "back street" practitioners. One alarming statistic highlighted by a reproductive healthcare study conducted in 2012, is that the number of induced abortions in Nigeria rose from 610,000 in 1996 to 1.2million in 2012. The lead author of the study surmised that 40% of women who engage in induced abortions suffer complications serious enough to require treatment. It is clear that there is significant scope for preventive measures in this area.

   Tubal blockage may also be due to a gynaecological condition called **Endometriosis**. The right fallopian tube may be blocked secondary to pelvic peritonitis arising from **inflammation of the appendix (Appendicitis).** If appendicitis is not diagnosed early and treated surgically, it can lead to rupture of the appendix which will lead to generalised peritonitis and blockage of both fallopian tubes.

2) **Ovulatory disorder** – This is the second commonest cause of female factor infertility. Common causes of failure of ovulation include:
   a) Polycystic Ovary Syndrome (PCOS)
   b) Overweight --   Body Mass Index (BMI) of 30 or higher
   c) Underweight – Body Mass Index (BMI) less than 19
   d) Stress
   e) Poor Diet

3) **Poor Sperm Quality** – this may be **low sperm count, poor sperm motility (sluggish sperm)** or **high proportion of sperm with abnormal shape (abnormal morphology)**. Possible causes for poor sperm quality include: a) **smoking** b) **excessive alcohol consumption** c) **Genital infection / Sexually transmitted diseases,** d) **poor diet** e) **toxic chemicals** f) **trauma / injury to the genitals,** g) **drug abuse.**

4) **Erectile & Ejaculatory problems** -- causes of these are many and varied. Common causes include: medical condition such as **diabetes mellitus, stress, alcohol abuse, excessive smoking.** This problem is often a great source of embarrassment for affected men who are often reluctant to admit to it in a clinical setting.

Chapter 3
Reproductive Health Education

This is about knowledge of some basic fertility facts to protect fertility and increase the chance of becoming pregnant. Conception takes place when a woman's egg is fertilised by a man's sperm. For this process to be successful both egg and sperm have to be of good quality, the egg has to be released into the fallopian tube, the fallopian tube has to healthy and patent (open), the sperm has to swim from the vagina, through the cervix, the uterine cavity and into the fallopian tubes, and the sperm has to penetrate into the egg, and finally the embryo (fertilised egg) has to implant in the uterine So it is immediately evident that there are many potential bottlenecks in the fertility physiology. Indeed, human fertility is inefficient.

The chance of a couple with no fertility problems becoming pregnant on a month to month basis is only 25%. A normal semen sample produced during sexual intercourse contains an average of 22million sperm with at least 40% swimming well. Yet it takes multiple sexual intercourse (ideally 2-3 times a week) over several months (average of 6 months) before one sperm fertilises one egg to achieve a pregnancy. Compare this with reproduction in some species where a single act of sexual intercourse gives rise to conception and birth of multiple offsprings!

Normal female monthly cycle is between 27 to 31 days. An egg is released around mid-cycle which is 13 to 16 days from the start of the last menstruation. The egg is fertilised within 12 to 24 hours of being released.

 At the risk of stating the obvious, the biology (basis) of male and female fertility are different.

A woman is born with a finite number of eggs in her ovaries (about half a million) akin to having a set amount of money in a deposit bank account. ***The difference though, is that while money in a bank account may yield interest and increase your deposit, the number of eggs in the ovaries does not increase, on the contrary it actually declines in quantity and quality with increasing age.*** This is the reason for the decline in female fertility with age. This decline in fertility kicks in in the mid-30s and becomes significant from 40 years age. Pregnancy rates are very low after 44 years even with fertility treatment. The male fertility system is centred within the testes where spermatozoa (sperm cells) are produced. The production and maturation of sperm within the testes (spermatogenesis) takes about 2 to 3 months and require a lower temperature, a few degrees below normal body temperature. This is why the testes are positioned in the scrotum, and not inside the body. The essence of spermatogenesis is that fresh sperm cells are produced every 2 to 3 months. Compare this with the female where a 35year old woman has eggs that are effectively 35years old! I say this to emphasise the difference in "design" and underline the disadvantages of undue delay in starting a family.

Chapter 4
Tackling the commonest cause of infertility

Blockage of the fallopian tubes is the commonest cause of infertility in Nigeria. Tubal blockage is often caused by pelvic inflammatory disease (PID) arising from results from either sexually transmitted infection or from complications following induced abortion. Common organisms underlying this condition include Gonorrhea and Chlamydia.

According to the World Health Organisation (WHO) an estimated 34 million women, predominantly from developing countries have infertility which resulted from maternal sepsis and unsafe abortion. This is certainly a serious situation that needs concerted action on the parts of individuals, organisations, healthcare regulators and government.
One alarming statistic from a study conducted in 2012 is that the number of induced abortions in Nigeria rose from 610,000 in 1996 to 1.2 million in 2012. The study stated that 40% of women who engaged in induced abortions suffer complications serious enough to require treatment. Worse still, complications secondary to botched abortions is a common cause of death of young women. Herein lies the scale of the problem.
Male genital tract infection can also affect male fertility. Repeated gonorrhoea or chlamydial infection can cause inflammation of the testes and epididymis (epididymo-orchitis) and subsequent scarring. Scarring can cause obstruction of the tubules within the testes and lead to low or no sperm count.

Prevention of genital tract infection in
women and men
Key points

Healthcare regulators must up their game and do everything possible to clamp down on poor practice and unqualified practitioners.

Government must play a lead role to galvanise the formulation of policies, provision of funds, enablement of agencies and organisations to facilitate the eradication of this nightmare scenario.

Chapter 5
Avoiding Risk factors

The risk factors are the same for both men and women. These are tabulated below:

Risk Factor	Comments
Age	A woman's fertility declines with age. Peak fertility occurs in the early to mid-twenties. Steady decline in fertility becomes noticeable from mid-thirties and from 40s fertility decline is significant. Therefore, it is unwise to unduly defer starting a family.
Weight	**12% of all infertility cases are caused because women either weigh too much or too little.** Being overweight adversely affects both female and male fertility. In women it mainly affects ovulation, egg quality and implantation. In men excessive body weight is correlated with poor sperm quality. In women being underweight affects ovulation negatively. Ideal Body Mass Index (BMI) is between 19 and 32.
Smoking	Nicotine and nicotine degradation products causes havoc with both egg and sperm quantity and quality. One mechanism through which smoking reduces male fertility is through increased toxic molecules (reactive oxygen species) which damages the sperm in more ways than is visible in routine semen analysis.
Alcohol consumption	Excessive alcohol consumption is detrimental to both female and male fertility. Alcohol abuse can

	suppress sperm production and is associated with erectile dysfunction. In women alcohol apart from reducing fertility can cause serious harm to the unborn baby.
Stress	Moderate and severe stress can impair fertility in both men and women. In women stress can affect ovulation and sexual activity. In men stress can cause difficulty in getting erection and/or ejaculation.
Exposure to chemicals and environmental toxic substances	Metals and Chemicals such as Lead, Paint, Solvents and Pesticides are detrimental to sperm production. Radiation is also very harmful to sperm production.
Drug abuse	Use of Heroin, Cannabis, cocaine and crack cocaine can inhibit ovulation and decrease sperm count and motility. They are associated with high risk of Pelvic inflammatory disease and HIV infection due to their association with risky sexual behaviour. Use of steroids & testosterone for body building by men can suppress sperm production.
Occupational Hazards	Certain occupations can affect fertility. Working with radiation or in the paint production can suppress sperm production. Long distance drivers are at risk of poor sperm quality because their testes are subjected to high temperatures which is not favourable to sperm production.

Chapter 6
Lifestyle changes to improve your chances of conceiving

Making positive lifestyle changes can increase the chances of conceiving. Some important points have been made under the previous sections. Other lifestyle changes to enhance your chance of conception include:

- **No smoking / No alcohol consumption**
- **Exercise regularly** but for women it is important to point out that exercises must not be too intense. Strenuous and intense exercises can be counterproductive in women because it provokes the secretion of some hormones that can suppress the ovaries. This is why some female athletes do not have regular periods. Examples of suitable exercise for women include gentle stretching, walking , and swimming for 30 minutes two to three times a week.
- **Diet** – the ideal fertility-boosting diet should be rich in fish and green vegetables and fruits. Carbohydrate intake should be controlled and restricted to small portions especially in women with ovulatory problems be to Polycystic Ovary Syndrome (PCO). You may need to consult with a dietician or nutritionist for advice and guidance.
- **Avoidance of tight underpants in men** which have the effect of increasing the temperature around the scrotum which in turn will affect the formation of sperm
- **Avoid self-medication** – some medications may adversely affect sperm formation or ovulation or suppress implantation. For example ibuprofen tablets common used as pain killers can supress thickening of the endometrium (lining inside the womb) which will in turn cause implantation failure.

Regular Health checks and prompt attention to medical problems

Regular health checks will detect medical conditions such as high blood pressure, diabetes mellitus, and thyroid disorder all of which can affect fertility and pregnancy. Early diagnosis will allow treatment and effective control of these conditions.

If undiagnosed and untreated, diabetes mellitus can reek havoc with body systems and organs. In men it affects the nerves in the body and cause a variety of symptoms including inability to have or sustain erection, as well as problems with ejaculation whereby semen produced during intercourse goes into the urinary bladder (retrograde ejaculation) instead of being released into the female vagina. In females, diabetes affects ovulation and implantation which lead to infertility and in some cases miscarriages and complicated pregnancy lead to death of the baby inside the womb. These are serious problems indeed and emphasise the need for regular medical check up and prompt treatment of disease conditions when detected.

Chapter 7
How to boost sperm quality

The three cardinal pillars on which fertility stand include ovulation, tubal patency and functionality, and sperm quality. It should be stressed however that these three tenets are intricately inter-related and dependent on several other bodily systems and functions, not least the endocrine glands & hormones. While there are clinical and laboratory tests to evaluate the status of these important keys to fertility, the tests are not without limitations. For example, the fact that a fallopian tube is patent (open, no blockage) does not necessarily mean it is functional. Infact the tubal mucosal lining and cilia may be damaged from a variety of causes. There are also limitations in the assessment of male fertility.

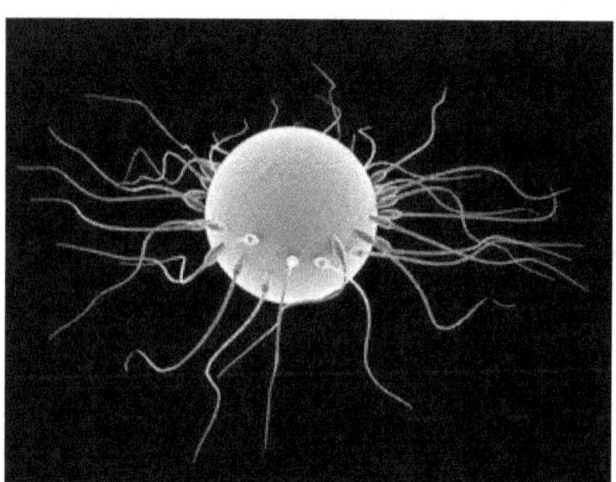

An analysis of cases of infertility shows 30% is due to a male factor, 30% to a female factor, 30% to a combination of both male and fertility, and 10% unexplained. The standard assessment of male fertility is through a semen analysis which has several limitations, including the well known sample to sample variation in any man. Therefore testing only one sample may not be truly representative of semen quality. It is good practice to carry out two semen tests 6 to 8 weeks apart.

Also, routine semen analysis does not test sperm function. The true test of sperm function is that which assesses the ability to fertilize an egg, but at present there isn't such a test in clinical practice.

New areas of research suggest that tests to assess degree of sperm DNA damage (Sperm DNA fragmentation test) may have clinical correlation to infertility and recurrent miscarriage.

Normal Semen Parameters – World Health Organisation Guidelines (WHO, 2010)

Parameter	Normal Values (WHO, 2010)
Semen volume (ml)	1.5 ml or more
Total sperm number (million per ejaculate)	39 million per ejaculate
Sperm concentration (million per ml)	15 million/ml or more
Progressive motility (%)	32% or more
Sperm morphology (normal forms, %)	4% or more
Vitality (live spermatozoa, %)	58% or more
White Blood Cells (million)	Less than 1million
Ph	≥ 7.2

It is important that even if the conventional semen analysis is "normal", the man should still take active measures to boost sperm quality. **There are several ways to improve your sperm quality**. The list below is comprehensive but not exhaustive. You should consider (with input from your partner) some of the approaches discussed below, write them down together with an action plan   this is your **Sperm Quality Improvement Plan (SQIP).**
Questions to ask your doctor about your sperm test report

1)Good explanation of your semen report: Don't be afraid, don't be shy, you should ask a point by point explanation of the report, ask about actual figures of the Volume, Liquefaction, Viscosity, sperm concentration, sperm motility, sperm morphology.
Ideally you want a copy of the report, actually seeing any suboptimal result might spur you on to determined corrective action

2) What are the likely causes of any subnormal result? The cause of abnormality in most sperm defects is often unclear and the subject of conjecture. However you should ask your doctor for his opinion on the possible causal factors which may help to focus on some particular corrective actions.

3) Is a clinical examination of the genitalia required? In some cases examination of the inguinal region, scrotum and testis may reveal some relevant factors such as varicocele, reduced testicular volume, and testicular tenderness

4) Do I need further tests, for example, repeat semen analysis, hormone levels, infection screen, chromosomes analysis? Some cases of sperm defects are due to hormonal problems e.g. a condition known as Hypogonadotrophic hypogonadism where the blood levels of FSH and LH are very low and there is no hormonal drive for sperm production (spermatogenesis). This condition is treatable with hormone replacement with FSH & LH injection. If there is any suggestion of infection in the semen, antibiotic treatment may be of help.

Strategies to improve Sperm Quality

1) General measures:

a) Get fit – regular exercises help but don't go overboard. Remember too much of a good thing may be bad.
b) Avoid tight fitting pants and trousers – these generate excessive high temperature around the scrotum and testes which suppress sperm production
c) Avoid hot baths
d) Replace your underpants with boxer shorts
e) Avoid self-medication
f) If you are trying for a pregnancy, regular sexual intercourse 2 to 3 times a week is effective. Long abstinence from sexual intercourse of more than 5 days may increase semen volume but sperm quality is reduced. This is one reason why it is not a good idea to restrict

intercourse to the woman's fertile period only. With regular sexual intercourse of 2-3 times a week there will be "a steady stream of sperm" within the female tract to fertilise an egg.

2) Lifestyle changes – these include:

a) **Stop smoking:** Nicotine and nicotine degradation products both suppress sperm production and damage the sperm cells already formed. It generates oxygen radicals (reactive oxygen species) which
are toxic to the sperm membrane. The sperm cells may look normal with good progressive motility but they would not be competent in fertilizing an egg. In other words you may be "firing blanks".
b) **NO** Alcohol
c) **DO NOT** use Recreational drugs
d) **DO NOT use anabolic steroids** used for body building

3) Weight reduction:
If you are overweight i.e. Body Mass Index (BMI) of 30 or more, you should start a weight reduction program. The program should include an exercise plan and dietary advice from your doctor or dietician.

4)Avoid Occupational / Environmental toxic substances such as
chemicals used in the paint industry and some insecticides

5) Fertility-enhancing diet: the Mediterranean diet consisting of
fish, green-vegetables, fruits are good for sperm production.

6)Vitamins & Minerals supplement: Vitamin C, E, Selenium are
well known anti-oxidants and will enhance sperm quality and function. **Folic acid tablets** are good for cell division and can enhance sperm production.

Sperm problems requiring specialist action
Some sperm problems are only amenable to specialist assessment
and remedies. One such example is *Azoospermia (absence of sperm
in semen).*

Azoospermia: This refers to absence of sperm in semen. This
requires examination of the testis as well as blood tests for
hormone levels including Follicle Stimulating Hormone (FSH),
Luteinising hormone (LH) and Testosterone level, to determine the
underlying cause. If the cause is hormonal then appropriate
hormone injections may be effective in stimulating sperm
production. If the cause is one of obstruction within the testes then
surgical sperm extraction is indicated and the retrieved sperm used
in treatment through a form of in vitro fertilisation called
intracytoplasmic injection (ICSI).
If tests indicate failure of testicular cells (called Sertoli cells) then
the treatment with donor sperm is the only option.

CONCLUSION

Infertility is a severe affliction on affected couples. Modern assisted reproductive technologies such as in vitro fertilisation (IVF) are effective treatment options but the high costs make them unaffordable for many couples. The commonest cause of infertility is blockage of fallopian tubes due in most cases to pelvic infection resulting from sexually transmitted infections and complication arising from induced abortions often carried out by unqualified and untrained practitioners in substandard premises. Clearly a lot can and should be done to prevent this sad scenario.

Individuals must take personal responsibility and action to preserve their reproductive health. Preservation of your fertility is your investment in the future of your lineage, your community and your nation.

As already discussed, prevention of infertility must include the following key strategies:

- Reproductive Health Education
- Tackling the commonest cause of infertility
- Avoiding risk factors for infertility
- Lifestyle changes
- Regular Health checks and prompt attention to any medical problem

And finally:

There ought to be local and national sensitization campaigns for prevention of infertility based on reproductive health education, fertility-boosting lifestyle habits, improved healthcare services, effective regulation of healthcare practitioners and premises to promote best practice and clamp down on untrained and unqualified charlatans dabbling in healthcare.

*All schools and colleges ought to offer **a course on Health Education** so that there is an awareness of what every individual can do to prevent certain health problems, eg obesity, diabetes, hypertension and infertility. This book should on the essential reading list for such a course.*

SUGGESTED READING

Centres for Disease Control and Prevention. National Public Health Action Plan for the Detection, Prevention and Management of Infertility. Atlanta, Georgia: Centres for Disease Control and Prevention; June 2014.

The Prevalence of Infertility & Its Preventive Measures in Sub-Saharan Africa. A presentation at the W.H.O, AFRO & EMRO Regional Management of Infertility Research. Professor R.J.I. Leke

JSI Research & Training Institute Inc./Denver. The future of Infertility Prevention Project Health Impact Assessment: Policy Implications and Recommendations in light of Passage of the Patient Protection & Affordable Care Act, July 25, 2012.

A review of Management of Infertility in Nigeria: framing the ethics of a national health policy. Published in International Journal of Women's Health. By Akinloye O, and Truter EJ, 2011.

www.ingramcontent.com/pod-product-compliance
Lightning Source LLC
Chambersburg PA
CBHW070023260726
48658CB00003B/1013